COMPLETE GUIDE TO BARRETT'S ESOPHAGUS

Navigating Allison-Johnstone Anomaly, Empowering Strategies For Diagnosis, Treatment, Lifestyle Management, Prevention, Care, And Long-Term Health

DEHART HAIRSTON

© [DEHART HAIRSTON], [2024]

All rights reserved. No part of this publication may be reproduced, distributed, or transmitted in any form or by any means, including photocopying, recording, or other electronic or mechanical methods, without the prior written permission of the publisher, except in the case of brief quotations embodied in critical reviews and certain other noncommercial uses permitted by copyright law.

DISCLAIMER

This book's content is only intended for general informative purposes. At the time of writing, the author has taken every precaution to guarantee that the material is correct and current. Nevertheless, the author disclaims all explicit and implicit representations and guarantees about the availability, appropriateness, correctness, completeness, and usefulness of the material on these pages.

Since the author is not a licensed medical practitioner, the material in this book shouldn't be interpreted as medical advice. Before making any modifications to their diet, exercise regimen, or medical treatment, readers are urged to speak with a licensed healthcare provider.

Moreover, the author has no connection to any of the businesses, organizations, or people that are discussed in this book. Any mentions of goods, services, businesses, or people are purely informative and do not indicate endorsement or suggestion.

This book's content is entirely dependent on the author's expertise, study, and comprehension of the topic. Despite having taken reasonable care to offer correct information, the author disclaims all liability for any mistakes or omissions in the material as well as for any losses, harm, or damages resulting from using the information.

It is recommended that readers use their own judgment and discretion when applying the knowledge in this book to their own situations. The use or implementation of any material in this book may result in unfavorable repercussions, directly or indirectly, for which the author assumes no liability.

By reading this book, you agree to release and hold the author harmless from any claims, losses, liabilities, costs, or expenditures resulting from or related to the use of the information you get from it.

Table of Contents

CHAPTER 1 13
- Understanding Barrett's Esophagus 13
- What Is Barrett's Esophagus? 13
- Causes And Risk Factors 14
  - 3. Gender: 15
  - 4. Obesity: 15
  - 6. Hiatal hernia: 15
- Symptoms And Signs 16
  - 5. Chronic cough: 16
  - 7. Unintentional weight loss: 17

CHAPTER 2 19
- Diagnosing Barrett's Esophagus 19
- Screening And Diagnosis Methods 19
- Importance Of Early Detection 21
- Talking To Your Doctor 22

CHAPTER 3 25
- Treatment Options 25
- Lifestyle Changes And Dietary Recommendations 25
- Medications For Managing Symptoms 27
  - Antacids: 28

- Prokinetics: 28
- Surgical Procedures And Interventional Therapies 28
  - Endoscopic Therapy: 29
  - Surgical Fundoplication: 29
- **CHAPTER 4** 31
  - Complications And Risks 31
  - Complications Associated With Barrett's Esophagus 31
  - Monitoring And Preventive Measures 33
  - Addressing Concerns And Anxiety 34
- **CHAPTER 5** 37
  - Living With Barrett's Esophagus 37
  - Coping Strategies And Emotional Support 37
  - Maintaining Quality Of Life 39
  - Building A Support Network 40
- **CHAPTER 6** 43
  - Diet And Nutrition 43
  - Foods To Include And Avoid 43
  - Meal Planning Tips 45
  - Importance Of Healthy Eating Habits 47
- **CHAPTER 7** 49

Managing Acid Reflux 49
Understanding Acid Reflux 49
Lifestyle Modifications For Acid Reflux 50
Over-The-Counter And Prescription Medications 51
CHAPTER 8 55
Doctor-Patient Communication 55
Effective Communication Strategies 55
   Active Listening: 55
   Ask Open-Ended Questions: 56
   Express Your Issues: 56
   Repeat Back Information: 56
   Use Plain Language: 57
   Take Notes: 57
   Follow-up: 57
Asking Questions And Seeking Clarifications 58
   Prepare ahead of time: 58
   Be precise: 58
   Don't Be hesitant to Ask for Clarifications: 58
   Ask About Alternatives: 59
   Seek Second Opinions if Necessary: 59
   Trust Your Instincts: 60

    Advocating For Your Health..................................60
        Be Proactive:...60
        Know Your Rights: 61
        Communicate Effectively: 61
        Bring a Support Person: 61
        Seek Second Opinions:.................................61
        Follow Through on Recommendations: 62
        Stay Informed:..62
CHAPTER 9 63
    Research And Advances 63
    Latest Research Findings 63
    Promising Treatments On The Horizon 65
    Participating In Clinical Trials 67
CHAPTER 10 71
    Prevention And Long-Term Outlook 71
    Preventive Measures For Barrett's Esophagus 71
    Long-Term Management Strategies.........................73
    Empowering Yourself Through Knowledge...........76
    CONCLUSION..78
THE END 81

ABOUT THIS BOOK

"Barrett's Esophagus" is more than just another medical book; it's a lifeline for anybody dealing with this ailment. In its pages, readers will get a thorough introduction to Barrett's Esophagus, from comprehending its intricacies to dealing with its complexity. Let me explain why this book is indispensable:

First, it clarifies Barrett's Esophagus. The first chapter sets the framework by defining it and outlining its causes, symptoms, and indicators. This fundamental knowledge is critical for anybody dealing with this disorder, whether they are patients, caregivers, or healthcare providers.

Chapter 2 focuses on diagnosing Barrett's Esophagus, emphasizing the necessity of early identification. Readers who understand screening procedures and the need to receive quick medical treatment may successfully advocate for their health.

Chapter 3 discusses treatment options, which include lifestyle modifications, medicines, and surgical treatments. This provides readers with options and prepares them to interact with their healthcare team to make educated decisions customized to their requirements.

Complications and dangers are unavoidable issues that are thoroughly covered in Chapter 4. Readers may take control of their health and reduce anxiety by learning about possible dangers and preventative steps.

Chapter 5 focuses on the emotional element, providing coping skills and emphasizing the need for support networks. This comprehensive approach recognizes the significant effect Barrett's Esophagus may have on a person's quality of life.

Diet and nutrition take center stage in Chapter 6, which offers practical advice on food selection and meal planning. These insights may help you maintain your general well-being and efficiently manage symptoms.

Chapter 7 delves further into managing acid reflux, a major side effect of Barrett's Esophagus. Readers are provided with strategies to alleviate suffering, including lifestyle changes and prescription alternatives.

Effective doctor-patient communication is essential, as stressed in Chapter 8. By developing a collaborative connection with their healthcare professionals, readers may manage their path with clarity and confidence.

Chapter 9 brings readers up to date on the newest research and therapy developments, allowing them to pursue promising routes and perhaps participate in clinical trials.

Finally, Chapter 10 focuses on preventive and long-term management, emphasizing the value of proactive efforts and offering hope for a better future.

In essence, "Barrett's Esophagus" is more than simply a book; it's a guidebook for empowerment and fortitude in the face of a difficult disease. It's a light of information, compassion, and support for everyone affected by Barrett's Esophagus, helping them to greater health and a more fulfilling life.

CHAPTER 1

Understanding Barrett's Esophagus

What Is Barrett's Esophagus?

Barrett's esophagus is a disorder in which the normal tissue lining the esophagus, the tube that links the mouth to the stomach, is replaced by tissue similar to that found in the intestine. This alteration happens as a consequence of persistent stomach acid exposure, which is often caused by gastroesophageal reflux disease (GERD). The illness is named after Dr. Norman Barrett, an Australian surgeon who originally characterized it in 1950.

The lining of the esophagus is normally made up of squamous epithelial cells that are flat and protective. However, in Barrett's esophagus, these cells are replaced with columnar epithelial cells that look like those seen in the intestines.

This alteration, known as metaplasia, is considered a pre-cancerous disease because it raises the chance of developing esophageal adenocarcinoma, which is a kind of cancer.

Causes And Risk Factors

Barrett's esophagus is mostly caused by chronic gastroesophageal reflux disease (GERD), a condition in which stomach acid and other contents flow backward from the stomach into the esophagus. Chronic exposure to stomach acid irritates and destroys the esophageal lining over time, resulting in the development of Barrett's esophagus in certain people.

Several risk factors raise the possibility of having Barrett's esophagus, including:

1. Chronic GERD is the key risk factor for Barrett's esophagus. Individuals with a lengthy history of GERD are more prone to acquiring this illness.

2. Barrett's esophagus is more frequent in older persons, especially those over the age of 50.

3. Gender: Men are more prone than women to develop Barrett's Esophagus.

4. Obesity: Being overweight, particularly around the belly, increases the chance of getting GERD and Barrett's esophagus.

5. Tobacco use may weaken the lower esophageal sphincter, the muscle valve that keeps stomach contents from returning to the esophagus, increasing the risk of GERD and Barrett's esophagus.

6. Hiatal hernia: A hiatal hernia occurs when a portion of the stomach protrudes through the diaphragm into the chest cavity, which may lead to GERD and Barrett's Esophagus.

Symptoms And Signs

Barrett's esophagus does not often produce symptoms. Instead, symptoms are often linked to gastroesophageal reflux disease (GERD), which is the primary cause of Barrett's esophagus in most instances. Common symptoms of GERD are:

1. Heartburn is a burning feeling in the chest that usually occurs after eating or when lying down.

2. Regurgitation is the reflux of sour fluid or food into the throat or mouth.

3. Dysphagia refers to difficulty swallowing, particularly solid meals.

4. Chest pain is discomfort or pain in the chest that may sometimes be mistaken for heart trouble.

5. **Chronic cough:** A chronic cough that is usually worse at night and may be caused by refluxed stomach acid hurting the throat.

6. Hoarseness is defined as a raspy or strained voice caused by stomach acid irritating the vocal cords.

7. **Unintentional weight loss:** Some people with severe GERD may lose weight owing to difficulties eating or pain when eating.

It's crucial to emphasize that not everyone with GERD develops Barrett's esophagus, and not everyone who has Barrett's esophagus develops esophageal cancer. Individuals with Barrett's esophagus, on the other hand, need continuous monitoring and therapy to identify any precancerous alterations early on and lower their chance of developing cancer.

CHAPTER 2

Diagnosing Barrett's Esophagus

Screening And Diagnosis Methods

Barrett's esophagus requires early identification. But how can physicians detect this condition? Healthcare practitioners use a variety of screening and diagnostic tools to diagnose and monitor Barrett's esophagus.

Upper endoscopy, also known as esophagogastroduodenoscopy (EGD), is a commonly used technique. A small, flexible tube with a camera attached to one end is inserted via the mouth and into the esophagus, stomach, and duodenum. This enables the clinician to physically evaluate the esophageal lining for any abnormalities, such as changes in color or texture, which might suggest Barrett's esophagus.

Tissue samples, known as biopsies, may also be collected during the process for subsequent examination under a microscope.

Another diagnostic technique is the barium swallow test, sometimes known as an esophagram. During this operation, the patient consumes a chalky beverage containing barium, which covers the esophageal lining and makes it visible on X-rays. X-ray pictures are then obtained while the barium goes down the esophagus, enabling the doctor to detect any abnormalities in the esophageal lining.

Furthermore, imaging methods such as endoscopic ultrasonography (EUS) may be utilized to determine the depth of any observed abnormalities and whether they have reached the deeper layers of the esophageal wall.

These screening and diagnostic approaches are critical for detecting Barrett's esophagus in its early stages, allowing for timely treatment and care to avoid problems like esophageal cancer.

Importance Of Early Detection

Early identification of Barrett's esophagus is critical for a variety of reasons. Barrett's esophagus is a precursor of esophageal adenocarcinoma, a disease that may be aggressive and difficult to cure if not detected early. By detecting Barrett's esophagus in its early stages, healthcare practitioners may take steps to lower the risk of cancer.

Furthermore, early discovery allows for proper monitoring and care of Barrett's esophagus, which may help patients avoid problems and achieve better results. Regular surveillance endoscopies may assist healthcare practitioners in tracking the evolution of the illness and detecting any changes that may signal an increased risk of cancer development.

Additionally, early discovery allows patients to make lifestyle adjustments and implement measures to successfully manage their illness. This may include dietary changes, weight control, and quitting smoking, all of which may help minimize the risk of disease development while improving general health.

Overall, early discovery of Barrett's esophagus allows healthcare practitioners to intervene more proactively, giving patients the greatest chance of treating their illness and lowering the risk of complications like esophageal cancer.

Talking To Your Doctor

If you feel you have Barrett's esophagus or are at risk because of persistent acid reflux or a family history of the ailment, you should see your doctor. Open communication with your healthcare physician is essential for prompt screening and diagnosis, as well as effective disease treatment.

When addressing your concerns with your doctor, offer a thorough medical history, including any symptoms you may be having, such as heartburn, trouble swallowing, or chest discomfort. In addition, tell your doctor about any risk factors you may have, such as obesity, smoking, or a history of gastrointestinal problems.

Depending on your symptoms and risk factors, your doctor may offer screening tests like an upper endoscopy or a barium swallow test. If Barrett's esophagus is identified, your doctor may work with you to create a treatment plan that is specific to your requirements, which may involve lifestyle changes, medication, or frequent surveillance endoscopies.

Remember that your doctor is there to assist you navigate the diagnosis and treatment of Barrett's esophagus, so don't be afraid to ask questions or seek clarification on any part of your care. By actively participating in talks with your healthcare practitioner, you may take charge of your health and strive toward optimal disease management.

CHAPTER 3

Treatment Options

Barrett's Esophagus is a disorder that requires care and treatment to avoid complications such as esophageal cancer. Treatment methods are intended to ease symptoms, manage the illness, and lower the risk of progression.

Lifestyle Changes And Dietary Recommendations

Making lifestyle and nutritional modifications may have a substantial influence on Barrett's Esophagus management. These adjustments are largely aimed at lowering acid reflux, which is a significant factor in the condition's development.

Dietary modifications may help reduce reflux and pain. Avoiding trigger foods, such as spicy, acidic, or fatty meals, may help to decrease esophageal inflammation.

Choosing smaller, more frequent meals over larger ones may also help reduce reflux attacks. Additionally, avoiding coffee, alcohol, and carbonated drinks might help with symptom control.

Elevating the Head of the Bed: Raising the head of your bed might prevent stomach acid from returning to the esophagus as you sleep. This simple change may reduce evening discomfort and improve sleep quality.

Weight Management: Maintaining a healthy weight is essential for treating Barrett's Esophagus. Excess weight exerts strain on the belly, worsening reflux symptoms. Regular exercise and proper eating habits may help with weight management and symptom control.

Smoking cessation: Smoking has been shown to aggravate acid reflux and raise the chance of Barrett's Esophagus problems.

Quitting smoking may greatly alleviate symptoms and lower the chance of disease development.

Medications For Managing Symptoms

Medications are essential for managing symptoms and avoiding complications from Barrett's Esophagus. Several drugs are routinely used to treat symptoms and lower acid production.

Proton Pump Inhibitors (PPIs): PPIs are drugs that inhibit the formation of stomach acid. They are often recommended to people with Barrett's Esophagus to relieve symptoms and prevent additional damage to the esophagus. PPIs may be purchased over the counter or at larger dosages with a prescription.

H2 Receptor Antagonists act by inhibiting histamine receptors in the stomach, lowering acid production. While not as strong as PPIs, they may nevertheless alleviate symptoms and are often used in combination with other drugs.

Antacids: Antacids are over-the-counter drugs that neutralize stomach acid and provide immediate but temporary relief from symptoms. They are often used to relieve occasional heartburn and reflux symptoms.

Prokinetics: These drugs promote esophageal motility and minimize the number of reflux episodes. They function by tightening the lower esophageal sphincter and facilitating gastric emptying, which reduces the amount of acid that runs back into the esophagus.

Surgical Procedures And Interventional Therapies

Lifestyle adjustments and drugs may not always be enough to alleviate symptoms or prevent disease development.

In such cases, surgical techniques and interventional therapy may be indicated to successfully treat Barrett's Esophagus.

Endoscopic Therapy: A flexible tube with a camera (endoscope) is used to treat Barrett's Esophagus and its complications. Radiofrequency ablation (RFA) and cryotherapy are two frequently used techniques for removing diseased tissue and promoting healthy tissue regeneration.

Surgical Fundoplication: Fundoplication is a surgical operation that includes wrapping the top of the stomach around the lower esophagus to strengthen the lower esophageal sphincter and reduce acid reflux. This surgery is normally reserved for those who haven't responded to medicines or endoscopic treatments.

Laparoscopic anti-reflux surgery, commonly known as Nissen fundoplication, is a minimally invasive technique designed to strengthen the lower esophageal sphincter and prevent acid reflux. During the surgery, the upper section of the stomach is wrapped around the lower esophagus, forming a valve-like system that keeps stomach acid from entering the esophagus.

Esophagectomy is a surgical surgery that removes a piece or all of the esophagus. It is used as a last resort therapy for severe instances of Barrett's Esophagus or when other treatments have failed. Esophagectomy has considerable risks and problems and is often reserved for late disease stages or instances of esophageal cancer.

Controlling Barrett's Esophagus requires a multifaceted strategy that includes lifestyle changes, drugs, and, in some circumstances, surgical treatments.

CHAPTER 4

Complications And Risks

Complications Associated With Barrett's Esophagus

Barrett's esophagus, although usually asymptomatic, may cause significant problems if left untreated. One of these complications is the development of esophageal cancer. The change of normal esophageal cells into those that resemble intestinal cells (intestinal metaplasia) raises the risk of cancer development. However, it is important to recognize that not everyone with Barrett's esophagus will get cancer. The risk varies from person to person, and variables such as age, gender, and the existence of other medical disorders may all impact it.

Another consequence of Barrett's esophagus is the development of dysplasia. Dysplasia is characterized by aberrant cell development and may vary from low to high grade. High-grade dysplasia is particularly concerning since it suggests a greater chance of malignant alterations in the esophagus tissue. Regular monitoring and surveillance of Barrett's esophagus is critical for detecting dysplasia early and intervening effectively to avoid cancer development.

Barrett's esophagus may cause additional issues than cancer and dysplasia, such as esophageal strictures. These esophageal narrowings may cause difficulties swallowing, chest discomfort, and even food impaction. Strictures are caused by prolonged inflammation and scarring of esophageal tissue. While not everyone with Barrett's esophagus develops strictures, there are possible consequences that must be managed and treated to ease symptoms and enhance quality of life.

Monitoring And Preventive Measures

Regular monitoring and surveillance are critical components in treating Barrett's esophagus and avoiding complications. The frequency and kind of monitoring are determined by various parameters, including the existence of dysplasia, the length of Barrett's segment, and individual risk factors. Individuals with Barrett's esophagus without dysplasia should have frequent endoscopic exams to check the health of the esophageal tissue and discover any alterations early.

An endoscopy involves inserting a flexible tube with a camera attached (endoscope) into the mouth and down the esophagus to see the lining and, if required, collect tissue samples (biopsies). These samples are analyzed under a microscope to detect dysplasia or malignant alterations. The frequency between surveillance endoscopies varies, but for those without dysplasia, it is usually every 3 to 5 years.

Those with dysplasia need more regular observation to watch for malignant development. High-grade dysplasia often requires more invasive treatments, such as endoscopic mucosal resection (EMR) or radiofrequency ablation (RFA), to remove or destroy aberrant tissue and lower the risk of cancer formation. These are minimally invasive procedures that may be performed during an endoscopy.

Addressing Concerns And Anxiety

Living with Barrett's esophagus may elicit worry and fear about the possibility of consequences, notably cancer. Individuals with Barrett's esophagus must have open and honest talks with their healthcare professionals regarding their illness, including risk factors and successful management strategies.

Education and knowledge are critical in resolving issues and minimizing anxiety associated with Barrett's esophagus. Understanding the illness, its possible implications and accessible treatment choices allows people to take an active part in their healthcare. Lifestyle changes such as maintaining a healthy weight, quitting smoking and excessive alcohol use, and controlling acid reflux symptoms may all help lower the risk of problems and improve overall health.

Individuals suffering from Barrett's esophagus may benefit greatly from support groups and online forums, which can provide both emotional and practical help. Connecting with people who have similar experiences may provide comfort and a feeling of belonging. Furthermore, obtaining professional counseling or therapy may help people deal with the worry and stress associated with their disease.

To summarize, while Barrett's esophagus can cause risks and complications, proactive management, regular monitoring, and lifestyle changes can significantly reduce the likelihood of negative outcomes. Individuals with Barrett's esophagus can navigate their condition with confidence and peace of mind if they stay informed, seek help, and work closely with their doctors.

CHAPTER 5

Living With Barrett's Esophagus

Coping Strategies And Emotional Support

Living with Barrett's Esophagus can present several physical and emotional challenges. Coping strategies and emotional support are essential for dealing with this condition. One of the first steps in coping is to comprehend the diagnosis and its implications. It is natural to feel a variety of emotions, including fear, anxiety, and frustration. Seeking help from healthcare professionals, support groups, or therapists can provide important guidance and coping strategies.

Mindfulness and stress-reduction techniques can also help manage the emotional burden of living with Barrett's Esophagus. Meditation, yoga, and deep breathing exercises can all help you relax and feel better emotionally. Furthermore, keeping a positive attitude and focusing on the aspects of life that bring you joy and fulfillment can be empowering.

Communication is an important aspect of dealing with Barrett's Esophagus. Openly discussing feelings and concerns with loved ones can lead to greater understanding and support. To ensure that the condition is properly managed, any physical symptoms or limitations must be communicated to healthcare providers.

Developing resilience is critical for navigating the challenges of Barrett's Esophagus. This includes adapting to change, looking for solutions to problems, and remaining optimistic about the future. Connecting with others who have had similar experiences can provide a sense of belonging and validation, reducing feelings of isolation.

Maintaining Quality Of Life

Maintaining a high quality of life while living with Barrett's Esophagus necessitates a multifaceted approach that considers both physical and emotional health. Prioritizing self-care is critical, as is following the recommended lifestyle changes and treatment plans prescribed by healthcare providers.

Diet plays an important role in treating Barrett's Esophagus symptoms and lowering the risk of complications. Avoiding trigger foods, such as spicy or acidic foods, as well as practicing portion control and eating smaller, more frequent meals, can help relieve symptoms like heartburn and reflux.

Regular exercise can also improve the quality of life for people with Barrett's esophagus. Physical activity not only improves overall health and well-being, but it can also help you maintain a healthy weight and alleviate symptoms like reflux.

Furthermore, prioritizing sleep hygiene is critical for managing symptoms and improving overall health. Establishing a consistent sleep schedule, developing a relaxing bedtime routine, and optimizing the sleep environment can all improve sleep quality and overall well-being.

Participating in activities that bring joy and fulfillment is another important aspect of maintaining a high quality of life with Barrett's Esophagus. Whether it's spending time with loved ones, pursuing hobbies and interests, or joining support groups, finding sources of happiness and fulfillment can improve overall well-being.

Building A Support Network

Individuals living with Barrett's Esophagus must establish a strong support network. This network may include healthcare providers, family members, friends, and others who understand and empathize with the condition's challenges.

Healthcare providers play an important role in the support network by providing medical advice, monitoring symptoms, and adjusting treatment plans as needed. Open communication and trust with healthcare providers are critical for successfully managing Barrett's Esophagus.

Family and friends can provide emotional and practical support as you navigate the daily challenges of living with Barrett's Esophagus. This could include assisting with household tasks, accompanying to medical appointments, or simply lending a listening ear during difficult times.

Participating in Barrett's Esophagus support groups or online communities can help you feel more at ease and connected. Sharing experiences, exchanging tips and advice, and providing encouragement can be extremely helpful in dealing with the condition.

Friends and family members should also be educated about Barrett's Esophagus to foster understanding and support. Providing information about the condition, its symptoms, and how it affects daily life can help loved ones provide more meaningful support.

Individuals with Barrett's Esophagus can feel empowered to navigate the challenges of their condition and maintain a fulfilling quality of life by establishing a strong support network that includes healthcare providers, family, friends, and peers.

CHAPTER 6

Diet And Nutrition

Foods To Include And Avoid

Barrett's esophagus can be managed effectively with dietary modifications. Understanding which foods to include and which ones to avoid is crucial for managing symptoms and promoting overall health.

Incorporating a variety of nutrient-rich foods into your diet is essential. Fresh fruits and vegetables, whole grains, lean proteins, and healthy fats should form the foundation of your meals. These foods provide essential vitamins, minerals, antioxidants, and fiber, which can help support a healthy digestive system and reduce inflammation in the esophagus.

Certain foods can exacerbate symptoms of Barrett's esophagus and should be limited or avoided altogether. Spicy foods, acidic foods and beverages (like citrus fruits, tomatoes, and coffee), fatty and fried foods, chocolate, and carbonated beverages can all trigger heartburn and worsen acid reflux. Alcohol and caffeine should also be consumed in moderation, as they can relax the lower esophageal sphincter and increase the risk of reflux.

Opting for smaller, more frequent meals throughout the day rather than big, heavier meals might help avoid overeating and lessen GERD symptoms. Additionally, eating slowly, chewing food thoroughly, and avoiding lying down immediately after eating can further reduce the likelihood of acid reflux.

Meal Planning Tips

Effective meal planning is crucial to keeping a balanced diet while controlling Barrett's esophagus. By making strategic decisions and planning meals, you can ensure that your diet promotes your general health and reduces discomfort.

Start by making a weekly meal plan that includes a range of nutritional meals. Focus on including lots of fruits and vegetables, whole grains, lean meats, and healthy fats in your meals and snacks. Experiment with new recipes and cooking techniques to keep meals interesting and pleasurable.

When planning your meals, consider your schedule and lifestyle. Choose fast and simple recipes for busy days and cook bigger amounts of meals that can be portioned up and stored for later use.

This may help you resist the lure of harmful convenience meals when you're short on time.

Be cautious of meal sizes and avoid overeating, since extra weight may worsen symptoms of Barrett's esophagus. Aim to fill half of your plate with veggies, one-quarter with lean protein, and one-quarter with nutritious grains or starchy vegetables. This balanced approach might help you feel content without overwhelming your digestive system.

Don't forget to remain hydrated by drinking lots of water throughout the day. While it's crucial to avoid extra drinks during meals to prevent diluting stomach acid, keeping hydrated between meals may assist in maintaining good digestion and lessen the risk of constipation.

Importance Of Healthy Eating Habits

Maintaining appropriate eating habits is vital for controlling Barrett's esophagus and boosting general well-being. By choosing good food choices and practicing mindful eating habits, you may minimize symptoms, encourage healing, and enhance your quality of life.

A balanced diet that includes a range of nutrient-rich foods delivers the vitamins, minerals, and antioxidants your body needs to operate efficiently. These nutrients help maintain a healthy immune system, decrease inflammation, and promote tissue healing, which is particularly essential for persons with Barrett's esophagus.

In addition to controlling symptoms, proper eating habits may also help avoid problems linked with Barrett's esophagus, such as esophageal cancer. By keeping a healthy weight, avoiding excessive alcohol use, and limiting intake of foods that worsen reflux, you may lower your chance of disease development.

Furthermore, practicing mindful eating techniques, such as eating slowly, digesting food fully, and paying attention to hunger and fullness signals, may help avoid overeating and lessen symptoms of acid reflux. By concentrating on the sensory experience of eating and listening to your body's cues, you may build a healthy connection with food and improve digestion.

Overall, adopting appropriate eating habits is critical for controlling Barrett's esophagus and enhancing long-term health results. By selecting good food choices, planning meals carefully, and practicing moderation, you may support your body's natural healing processes and have a higher quality of life.

CHAPTER 7

Managing Acid Reflux

Understanding Acid Reflux

Acid reflux, commonly known as gastroesophageal reflux disease (GERD), is a disorder where stomach acid rushes back into the esophagus, causing irritation and occasionally injury. The esophagus is the tube that delivers food from your mouth to your stomach, and when the lower esophageal sphincter (LES) – a muscle ring at the bottom of the esophagus – doesn't seal correctly, the acid may splash up into the esophagus. This may lead to symptoms including heartburn, regurgitation, chest discomfort, and trouble swallowing.

Understanding the processes underlying acid reflux may empower people to take control of their disease.

It's crucial to remember that occasional acid reflux is normal, but frequent or severe symptoms may indicate GERD, which needs therapy to avoid problems including Barrett's esophagus and esophageal cancer.

Lifestyle Modifications For Acid Reflux

Lifestyle adjustments are frequently the first line of defense in treating acid reflux. Simple modifications in everyday activities may drastically lessen symptoms and enhance quality of life. Dietary modifications play a significant part - avoiding trigger foods like spicy, acidic, or fatty meals may help lessen reflux episodes. Additionally, eating smaller, more frequent meals rather than big ones might aid digestion and lessen the incidence of reflux.

Maintaining a healthy weight is vital, since extra belly fat may put pressure on the stomach and increase acid symptoms. Elevating the head of the bed while sleeping may help prevent acid from leaking into the esophagus throughout the night. This may be performed by putting blocks beneath the bedposts or utilizing a wedge cushion.

Avoiding tight clothes, particularly around the waist, helps relieve pressure on the stomach and LES, minimizing the incidence of acid reflux. Smoking and excessive alcohol use may also weaken the LES and increase acid production, therefore quitting smoking and reducing alcohol intake are key lifestyle modifications for controlling GERD.

Over-The-Counter And Prescription Medications

In addition to lifestyle improvements, drugs may give relief from acid reflux symptoms and help avoid problems like Barrett's esophagus. Over-the-counter antacids like Tums or Rolaids may neutralize stomach acid and give rapid relief from heartburn. However, they are not meant for long-term usage and may not be adequate for treating more severe symptoms.

Histamine-2 receptor antagonists (H2 blockers) and proton pump inhibitors (PPIs) are routinely recommended drugs for GERD. H2 blockers function by lowering the generation of stomach acid, whereas PPIs are more strong and effectively stop acid production. These drugs may give long-lasting comfort and help cure esophageal damage caused by reflux.

It's crucial to utilize drugs as advised by a healthcare expert and to be aware of any adverse effects and interactions. While over-the-counter drugs may be beneficial for occasional symptoms, persistent GERD may need prescription-strength medication or other therapies.

In summary, controlling acid reflux entails a mix of lifestyle adjustments and drugs to minimize symptoms and avoid problems like Barrett's esophagus. Individuals who understand the causes of reflux and follow suitable treatments might regain control of their disease and improve their quality of life. Regular contact with a healthcare practitioner is required for tailored treatment and continuing support.

CHAPTER 8

Doctor-Patient Communication

Effective Communication Strategies

Communication between physicians and patients is critical for providing successful treatment. Establishing a solid connection with your healthcare professional may result in greater understanding, trust, and, ultimately, better health results. Here are some good communication strategies:

Active Listening: When discussing your health issues with your doctor, you should actively listen to what they have to say. This entails paying full attention, keeping eye contact, and avoiding distractions. Active listening allows you to better grasp your doctor's advice and ask pertinent questions.

Ask Open-Ended Questions: Rather than asking yes or no questions, attempt to encourage your doctor to give extensive responses. Instead of asking, "Is this treatment safe?" consider asking, "What are the potential risks and benefits of this treatment?"

Express Your Issues: Don't be afraid to discuss your issues, anxieties, or doubts with your doctor. Your healthcare professional is there to help you, but they can only address your problems if they understand what they are. Be upfront and honest about how you're feeling, both physically and emotionally.

Repeat Back Information: To ensure that you comprehend the information supplied by your doctor, try repeating it back to them in your own words. This helps you to explain any ambiguities and ensure that you have a thorough picture of the issue.

Use Plain Language: Medical jargon may be perplexing, so don't be hesitant to ask your doctor to clarify things in layman's terms. They should be able to explain difficult medical topics in a manner that you can grasp.

Take Notes: Taking notes during visits might help you recall critical information later. You might also ask your doctor whether it's acceptable to record the talk and go back to it later.

Follow-up: If you have any questions or concerns after your visit, please do not hesitate to contact your doctor. You may book a follow-up appointment or contact us by phone or email.

By using these communication tactics, you may establish a strong rapport with your doctor and guarantee that you get the best possible treatment.

Asking Questions And Seeking Clarifications

Asking questions and requesting clarification are critical components of efficient communication between patients and physicians. Here's how to properly participate in this process:

Prepare ahead of time: Before your meeting, take some time to jot down any questions or concerns you may have. This guarantees that you don't forget anything during your session and keeps you focused on what's most essential.

Be precise: Ask inquiries that are as precise as possible. Instead of asking a general question like, "What can I do to improve my health?" try something more specific like, "What dietary changes can I make to lower my cholesterol?".

Don't Be hesitant to Ask for Clarifications: If you don't understand anything your doctor says, don't be hesitant to seek clarification.

Your doctor is there to assist you, and they want to ensure that you understand your medical condition and treatment choices.

Write down your doctor's replies to your inquiries. This helps you remember the material and provides something to go back to if you have any more questions.

Ask About Alternatives: If your doctor advises a certain therapy or plan of action, don't be afraid to inquire about other possibilities. Your doctor should be able to explain the advantages and disadvantages of various techniques, allowing you to make an educated choice.

Seek Second Opinions if Necessary: If you are uncertain about your doctor's suggestion or diagnosis, do not be afraid to seek a second opinion. It's your health, and you have the right to consider other solutions and opinions.

Trust Your Instincts: You know your body better than anybody else. If something doesn't seem right or you're not sure about your doctor's opinion, follow your instincts and seek more help.

You may obtain a better awareness of your health condition and make more educated choices about your treatment if you actively communicate with your doctor and ask pertinent questions.

Advocating For Your Health

Advocating for your health entails taking an active role in healthcare choices and ensuring that your needs and preferences are met. Here are some ideas to advocate for your health:

Be Proactive: Take an active part in your healthcare by learning about your ailment and available treatments. Ask questions, gather knowledge, and take an active role in your health.

Know Your Rights: As a patient, you have the right to informed consent, privacy, and access to your medical records. Don't be afraid to express your rights if you believe they are being infringed.

Communicate Effectively: Explain your requirements, concerns, and preferences to your healthcare professionals. Be honest and upfront about your symptoms, lifestyle behaviors, and any other pertinent information that might assist guide your treatment.

Bring a Support Person: If you are feeling overwhelmed or scared by medical visits, try bringing a trusted friend or family member with you for support. They may assist you ask questions, take notes, and provide emotional support.

Seek Second Opinions: If you're uncertain about a diagnosis or treatment plan, don't be afraid to seek a second opinion from another healthcare professional. Before making significant healthcare choices, you should consider all of your alternatives and views.

Follow Through on Recommendations: Once you and your doctor have decided on a treatment plan, be sure you adhere to their recommendations. This involves taking prescribed drugs, attending follow-up visits, and implementing any necessary lifestyle modifications.

Stay Informed: Learn about medical developments and new treatment options for your disease. Knowledge is power, and being educated may help you make the greatest choices for your health.

By advocating for your health and actively engaging in your healthcare choices, you can guarantee that you get the finest treatment available and reach your health goals.

CHAPTER 9

Research And Advances

Latest Research Findings

Barrett's esophagus, a disorder in which the esophageal lining changes, is an ongoing study topic. Scientists and medical experts are always working to improve their knowledge of the disorder, including its origins, development, and possible therapies. One of the most recent study results concerns the molecular pathways that underpin the development of Barrett's esophagus. Researchers hope to discover new targets for medicines and interventions by examining the various biological processes and genetic elements involved.

Furthermore, advances in imaging methods have allowed for more accurate diagnosis and surveillance of Barrett's esophagus.

High-definition endoscopes and sophisticated imaging modalities, such as confocal laser endomicroscopy (CLE), provide comprehensive images of esophageal tissue, allowing for early diagnosis and evaluation of the problem. These advances not only improve diagnostic accuracy but also help guide therapy choices.

Another prominent area of study is the function of inflammation and the immune system in Barrett's esophagus. Chronic inflammation is thought to contribute to the development of the disease to esophageal cancer. Researchers hope to create tailored medicines that may reduce inflammation and slow disease progression by better understanding the inflammatory pathways and immune responses involved.

Furthermore, genetic and molecular investigations have shown a hereditary propensity to Barrett's esophagus and its consequences.

Identifying precise genetic markers linked with an elevated risk of acquiring the illness enables more individualized risk assessment and early intervention measures. Furthermore, knowing the molecular pathways that drive the transition of normal esophageal cells into Barrett's epithelium offers the potential for developing new preventative and therapeutic strategies.

Promising Treatments On The Horizon

In recent years, tremendous progress has been achieved in the development of innovative Barrett's esophagus therapies. One potential option is endoscopic treatment, which tries to remove or ablate aberrant tissue in the esophagus. Radiofrequency ablation (RFA), cryotherapy, and endoscopic mucosal resection (EMR) are less invasive alternatives to typical surgical treatments, allowing for tailored treatment with lower risk and recovery time.

Furthermore, the advent of precision medicine has opened the path for individualized treatment regimens based on each patient's genetic profile and illness features. Targeted therapeutics targeting particular molecular pathways involved in the etiology of Barrett's esophagus have enormous promise for enhancing treatment results and lowering the risk of progression.

Immunotherapy, which uses the immune system to target and remove malignant cells, is emerging as a viable therapeutic option for Barrett's esophagus and related esophageal cancers. Immunotherapeutic drugs, which modulate immune responses and improve immune surveillance, provide fresh hope to patients with advanced or resistant illnesses.

Furthermore, research studies are underway to assess the effectiveness of new treatment drugs, combination therapy, and preventative strategies in

Barrett's esophagus patients. Participation in these studies not only gives patients access to cutting-edge medicines but also helps to expand scientific understanding and create future standards of care.

Participating In Clinical Trials

Clinical trials are critical in expanding medical knowledge and improving patient outcomes in Barrett's esophagus. Patients who participate in clinical trials have the chance to get breakthrough treatments and contribute to the discovery of new remedies for the ailment. Clinical trials may assess the effectiveness and safety of new medications, surgeries, or treatment approaches in various stages of Barrett's esophagus, from early illness to advanced esophageal cancer.

Before entering in a clinical trial, participants are evaluated thoroughly to determine their eligibility and appropriateness for the study.

This assessment consists of a comprehensive medical history review, physical examination, diagnostic testing, and screening procedures. Patients also get full information on the clinical trial's goal, procedures, possible dangers, and benefits, allowing them to make educated choices regarding their participation.

A diverse team of healthcare professionals, including doctors, nurses, and research coordinators, closely supervises and monitors patients during the clinical study. Throughout the experiment, there are regular follow-up visits and evaluations to evaluate treatment response, monitor for adverse events, and maintain patient safety.

Furthermore, clinical trials are conducted by ethical standards and regulatory criteria to safeguard participants' rights, safety, and well-being. IRBs and regulatory authorities examine and approve clinical trial protocols to guarantee scientific rigor, patient safety, and ethical compliance.

Patients who participate in clinical trials not only receive access to potentially useful medications but also help to advance medical knowledge and find novel remedies for Barrett's esophagus. Their participation is critical to research initiatives aimed at improving the results and quality of life for people living with this illness.

CHAPTER 10

Prevention And Long-Term Outlook

Preventive Measures For Barrett's Esophagus

Understanding the risk factors for Barrett's Esophagus and taking proactive efforts to reduce them is the first step in preventing it. Chronic gastroesophageal reflux disease (GERD) is a major risk factor, thus treating it efficiently is critical for prevention. This often entails lifestyle adjustments such as maintaining a healthy weight, avoiding reflux-causing foods (such as hot or fatty foods), and eating smaller, more frequent meals to relieve strain on the esophageal sphincter.

Additionally, stopping smoking and limiting alcohol use may help avoid Barrett's Esophagus. Both smoking and drinking may weaken the lower esophageal sphincter, making it easier for stomach acid to flow back into the esophagus. Individuals may drastically reduce their risk by removing or changing these practices.

Regular screening and monitoring are also important preventative strategies, particularly for those with a history of GERD or other risk factors. Routine endoscopies enable physicians to identify any abnormalities in the esophagus early on, perhaps detecting Barrett's Esophagus before it evolves to a more advanced stage of cancer.

Maintaining overall good health via regular exercise, a nutritious diet rich in fruits and vegetables, and stress management may all help to avoid Barrett's Esophagus. These lifestyle choices not only promote digestive health but also boost the immune system, possibly lowering the risk of inflammation and cellular alterations in the esophagus.

To summarize, avoiding Barrett's Esophagus requires a multimodal strategy that includes successfully controlling GERD, adopting a healthy lifestyle, getting frequent screenings, and being aware of specific risk factors.

Long-Term Management Strategies

Once identified with Barrett's Esophagus, long-term treatment is critical to avoiding complications and progression to esophageal cancer. Long-term therapy aims to minimize acid reflux and inflammation in the esophagus while keeping an eye out for evidence of dysplasia or malignant alterations.

Medication, particularly proton pump inhibitors (PPIs), which assist in lower stomach acid production, is a key component of long-term therapy. PPIs may ease GERD symptoms while lowering the risk of future esophageal damage. However, it is critical to utilize these drugs under the supervision of a healthcare expert, since long-term usage may cause adverse effects that need frequent examination.

In addition to medicine, lifestyle changes play an important role in long-term treatment. This includes avoiding trigger foods, keeping a healthy weight, raising the head of the bed to reduce nocturnal reflux, and giving up smoking. These adjustments may help to prevent reflux episodes and the risk of consequences.

Regular monitoring of endoscopies is an important part of long-term treatment. These treatments enable clinicians to check the esophagus for evidence of dysplasia or malignant alterations. The frequency of surveillance endoscopies is determined by individual risk factors and the existence of dysplasia.

Early diagnosis of aberrant cell alterations may result in more effective therapies and improved results.

In certain circumstances, sophisticated techniques such as radiofrequency ablation (RFA) or endoscopic mucosal resection (EMR) may be advised to eliminate aberrant tissue and lower the risk of cancer formation. These procedures are often done by gastroenterologists who specialize in treating Barrett's Esophagus.

Overall, long-term therapy of Barrett's Esophagus requires a multifaceted strategy that includes medication, lifestyle changes, frequent observation, and, if required, sophisticated therapies to avoid problems and ensure the best possible result for patients.

Empowering Yourself Through Knowledge

Empowering oneself via information is an essential component of successfully managing Barrett's Esophagus. Understanding the ailment, its risk factors, and treatment techniques enables people to actively participate in their healthcare journey and make educated choices.

Educational resources, support groups, and credible websites may all give useful information regarding Barrett's Esophagus, including symptoms, treatment choices, and lifestyle changes. Engaging with healthcare providers and asking questions during consultations may also assist in clearing up any confusion and ensure that patients have a thorough grasp of their ailment and its treatment.

Furthermore, keeping note of symptoms, food triggers, and drug efficacy might help people manage their illness daily.

Maintaining open contact with healthcare practitioners and quickly reporting any changes or concerns will help to ensure early treatments and avert consequences.

Individuals with Barrett's Esophagus may improve their quality of life while also lowering their risk of illness development by being educated and proactive. Empowering oneself with information not only enhances self-management but also promotes a feeling of control and confidence in negotiating the intricacies of life with a chronic illness.

CONCLUSION

Barrett's esophagus is a disorder in which the esophageal lining changes, usually as a result of long-term gastroesophageal reflux disease (GERD). It is a serious worry since it may result in esophageal adenocarcinoma. Several major themes emerge as we conclude our investigation of Barrett's esophagus.

To begin, early identification and treatment of Barrett's esophagus are critical in preventing cancer from developing. Individuals with Barrett's esophagus should have regular surveillance endoscopies with biopsies to check for dysplasia or early symptoms of malignancy.

Second, lifestyle changes are critical to controlling Barrett's esophagus and GERD. These may include dietary adjustments, weight reduction, raising the head of the bed, and avoiding particular trigger foods and behaviors.

Third, medicinal therapies such as proton pump inhibitors (PPIs) or H2 receptor antagonists are often administered to alleviate acid reflux and protect the esophageal lining. In certain circumstances, surgical operations may be required to reinforce the lower esophageal sphincter or remove damaged tissue.

Furthermore, continuing research aims to better understand the underlying causes of Barrett's esophagus and create more effective therapies. This involves researching genetic variables, the impact of inflammation, and discovering new treatment targets.

To summarize, Barrett's esophagus is the result of a complex interaction between genetic predisposition, lifestyle variables, and environmental effects.

Its treatment requires a collaborative effort combining gastroenterologists, pathologists, oncologists, and patients themselves. We may work to lessen the burden of esophageal adenocarcinoma linked with Barrett's esophagus by emphasizing early identification, adopting lifestyle changes, and developing new therapies. Vigilance, education, and continued research are critical in battling this disorder and improving the results for those afflicted.

THE END

www.ingramcontent.com/pod-product-compliance
Lightning Source LLC
Chambersburg PA
CBHW070316230526
45470CB00002B/902